the cold water therapy book

A Comprehensive Guide to Cold Water Immersion, Ice Baths, and Showers for Improved Health, Recovery, Mental Resilience, Sleep Quality, and Enhanced Immune System

hunter hazelton

life level up books, llc

The Cold Water Therapy Book: A Comprehensive Guide to Cold Water Immersion, Ice Baths, and Showers for Improved Health, Recovery, Mental Resilience, Sleep Quality, and Enhanced Immune System

Copyright © 2023 by Hunter Hazelton

Copyright © 2023 by Life Level Up Books, LLC

contents

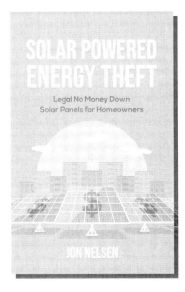

introduction

· · ·

WELCOME to The Cold Water Therapy Book: A Comprehensive Guide to Cold Water Immersion, Ice Baths, and Showers for Improved Health, Recovery, Mental Resilience, Sleep Quality, and Enhanced Immune System. If you're looking for a way to improve your physical health, mental resilience, sleep quality, and immune system, you've come to the right place. Cold water therapy has been around for centuries and has been known to have numerous benefits. It's a simple, yet effective practice that can help you feel better both physically and mentally.

IN THIS BOOK, we'll dive deep into the science behind cold water therapy and explore the techniques and best practices for mastering the art of cold water immersion. We'll also take a closer look at the benefits of cold water therapy for physical health, mental resilience, sleep quality, and immune system.

· · ·

WHETHER YOU'RE a beginner or an experienced cold water therapy enthusiast, this book has something for everyone. We'll cover everything from getting started with cold showers to safely integrating cold water therapy into your fitness routine. We'll even explore how to combine cold water therapy with other holistic health practices like meditation and yoga.

So, get ready to unlock the benefits of cold water therapy and make it a lifestyle. Let's dive in!

the science behind cold water therapy

. . .

How It Affects Your Body and Mind

COLD WATER THERAPY, an extraordinary adventure that holds the power to invigorate both body and mind. As you brave the chill, you might wonder if this is more than a refreshing dip. Is there something transformative about this seemingly extreme health tactic? Well, the answer lies in the fascinating science behind it.

As you submerge into cold water, your body is challenged by a form of controlled stress. Like an intense workout, it forces your body to react, adapt, and ultimately, become resilient. This triggers vasoconstriction, a process where blood vessels near the skin's surface contract, acting as a thermal blanket, safeguarding your vital organs against the cold.

When these blood vessels contract, your circulation accelerates, ensuring an efficient delivery of oxygen and nutrients. Imagine a fleet of delivery trucks, speeding through the city to meet its demands. The result? Lower inflammation, faster muscle recovery, and a strengthened immune system as your body rises to the challenge.

Now, let's shift our focus to the mind. The moment you plunge into cold water, your brain releases a surge of adrenaline and cortisol, steeling your body against the icy onslaught. This adrenaline rush, akin to an electric jolt, fills you with an enduring vitality.

· · ·

Moreover, cold water exposure can stimulate the production of dopamine and serotonin, the neurotransmitters that regulate mood and enhance overall wellbeing. It's as though your brain conducts a biochemical orchestra that not only diminishes stress and anxiety, but also instills a deep sense of focus and mental clarity. Like the chill sweeping away the cobwebs, your mind feels refreshed and sharp.

However, like all things, cold water therapy has its critics. They argue that the perceived benefits might be a placebo effect, where believing in the therapy's effectiveness creates a self-fulfilling prophecy. Critics also caution against potential hazards, such as hypothermia, cold water shock, or exacerbated medical conditions.

Yet, advocates of cold water therapy point to robust scientific research and countless testimonials from those who have experienced its transformative effects. They argue that, when used sensibly and under proper supervision, cold water therapy can be a safe and beneficial tool for overall wellness.

As you navigate the vast sea of information about cold water therapy, you'll encounter both skeptics cautioning about unseen dangers, and supporters cheering you on to discover the thrilling benefits for yourself. The ultimate choice rests with you, but it's undeniable that venturing into the icy depths of cold water therapy equips you with a wealth of knowledge and experience.

. . .

THE SCIENCE behind cold water therapy is as invigorating as it is fascinating. As you brave the chilly waters, you're embarking on more than just a swim. You're immersing yourself in a journey toward a healthier body and a sharper mind. So, dare to take the plunge and explore the refreshing benefits of cold water therapy for yourself.

getting started with cold showers

. . .

Tips for Beginners

EMBRACE the invigorating world of cold showers and unlock a treasure trove of benefits for your body and mind. If the idea of stepping under a frosty stream of water sends shivers down your spine, rest assured, with the right approach and a dash of courage, you too can experience the transformative effects of cold showers. Let's turn down the temperature and dive into the best advice on getting started!

BEGIN WITH A GENTLE DIP, not a bold plunge. Think of it like acclimatizing to the ocean. You don't dive in headfirst; you ease in, giving your body time to adapt. Start with your usual warm shower, then gradually reduce the temperature every 30 seconds or so. This gradual approach acclimatizes your body and mind to the new sensation, making the cold more manageable over time.

BREATHE, don't gasp. When the chilly water hits your skin, your body will instinctively gasp for air. But by practicing deep, controlled breathing, you can master this reaction. Picture yourself as a seasoned yogi, using each breath to maintain calm and focus amidst the icy challenge. This conscious breathing delivers more oxygen to your body, helping not only to keep you calm but also to enhance the benefits of your cold shower.

FIND YOUR WHY. Just like a climber embarking on a challenging climb, it's crucial to have a clear goal in mind. Pinpoint your reasons for embracing cold showers and the outcomes you hope to achieve. This purpose will guide you through moments of discomfort and doubt. Jot down these goals, keep them visible, and regularly remind yourself of them, especially when you're tempted to crank up the heat.

COMMIT TO A ROUTINE. Just like any physical training, consistency is key to reap the benefits of cold showers. Imagine you're training for a marathon; sporadic runs won't get you to the finish line. Develop a routine and adhere to it strictly. Start with a manageable step, like committing to a daily cold shower for one week. As you grow more comfortable, incrementally increase the duration and frequency until cold showers become a natural part of your routine.

ACKNOWLEDGE THE CHALLENGE. Cold showers can be uncomfortable, but it is in this discomfort that their therapeutic power lies. Envision yourself as a brave warrior entering a challenging battle. Embrace the difficulty and celebrate your victories, no matter how small. With each cold shower, you are cultivating mental toughness, resilience, and a sense of achievement that can translate into other areas of your life.

HOWEVER, it's essential to remember that cold showers aren't for everyone. For some people, particularly those with existing health conditions, cold showers can be overly strenuous or even risky. Always consult with your doctor before embarking on this frosty adventure and always listen to your body. Your primary goal should be self-care.

. . .

Additionally, manage your expectations. While cold showers offer numerous benefits, they aren't a magical cure-all. View them as one piece of a comprehensive wellness puzzle that also includes regular exercise, a balanced diet, and effective stress management techniques.

To wrap it up, initiating your cold shower practice is akin to boarding a thrilling roller coaster. There will be moments of anticipation, exhilaration, and perhaps a touch of apprehension. But with the right mindset, a gradual approach, and a commitment to consistency, you can harness the power of cold showers to transform your body and mind. So take a deep breath, embrace the challenge, and let the icy waves cascade over you, opening up a new realm of invigorating opportunities.

mastering the art of cold water immersion

. . .

Techniques and Best Practices

ARE you ready to dive into the intriguing realm of mastering cold water immersion? Submerging yourself into an icy bath can seem daunting, but with the right guidance and a sprinkle of courage, you too can unlock the amazing benefits this practice has to offer for both your mind and body.

CHOOSING the right environment for your icy plunge is as important as selecting the perfect venue for an unforgettable concert. You have options ranging from natural bodies of water like lakes and oceans, to man-made ice baths and cold plunge pools. Each presents unique challenges and benefits. So, explore different settings and find one that resonates with you. Prioritize your safety! Make sure your chosen location is safe and suitable for cold water immersion.

PREPARATION of both mind and body is key before stepping into the frigid waters. Think of yourself as a concert pianist, warming up your fingers before a performance. Engage in light physical activity to elevate your heart rate and warm up your muscles. Deep breathing exercises or meditation can help calm your nervous system and focus your mind on the task at hand.

BREATHING, during your icy dip, will serve as your anchor to reality. Fine-tune your breathing technique, as a seasoned diver would, to maintain control and composure. One popular method is the Wim Hof Method, which combines deep, regulated breathing with gradual exposure to cold.

Experiment with different techniques to find the one that suits you best.

GRADUAL EXPOSURE IS KEY. Just as you would when learning a new musical instrument, start slow and build up. Begin by immersing smaller body parts like your hands and feet, and over time, work your way up to full immersion. As your cold tolerance grows, so will your confidence and proficiency in the practice.

SET time limits and monitor your progress: Create clear boundaries for your cold water immersion sessions to ensure safety and track progress. Document your starting point, the duration of each session, and any physical or psychological changes you experience, much like an astronaut logging data for a mission report. This record will be invaluable for charting your progress and refining your cold water immersion technique.

WHILE THE BENEFITS of cold water immersion are compelling, it's crucial to approach this practice with a balanced perspective, just as a seasoned sommelier would when assessing a new wine. Cold water immersion might not be suitable for those with compromised immune systems or pre-existing health conditions. Always consult a healthcare professional before embarking on this frosty endeavor.

· · ·

PATIENCE, tolerance, and persistence are required to master cold water immersion. Don't expect immediate results or miraculous transformations. Instead, view your progress as a series of small victories that inch you closer to your ultimate goal.

EMBRACING the art of cold water immersion is like becoming a skillful surfer. It involves effort, persistence, and a willingness to step outside of your comfort zone. As you refine your techniques and adopt best practices, you will unlock a world of unparalleled benefits for your mind and body. So, wax your board, plot your course, and set sail on the thrilling voyage of mastering cold water immersion!

the benefits of cold water therapy for physical health

. . .

Pain Relief, Improved Circulation, and Recovery

ALTHOUGH THE ACT of submerging yourself in frigid water may initially appear intimidating, the benefits for your physical health make the chill worthwhile. Cold water therapy can assist your body in a variety of ways, from pain reduction to better circulation and healing. So let's discover the mysteries of this energizing workout by plunging into the icy depths!

Understanding the Benefits of Cold Water Therapy for Relieving Pain and Inflammation

IMAGINE LIVING in a society where pain and inflammation can be reduced without the need of drugs. You can do that with the use of cold water therapy. Your blood vessels contract when you submerge yourself in freezing water, decreasing blood flow to the injured area. This tightening can reduce swelling and pain in the muscles and joints. Additionally, the cold water may temporarily relieve pain by numbing the nearby nerves. But it's crucial to keep in mind that cold water therapy is not a cure-all for all forms of pain, just like with any natural medication. Before adopting cold water therapy into your regimen, it's imperative to get medical guidance if you feel chronic or intense pain.

Increasing Circulation and Oxygenation: Cold Water Therapy's Physical Advantages

Your circulatory system drives your body by transporting nutrients and oxygen to your cells while eliminating waste products from them. Your circulation can be helped with cold water therapy, which can help your muscles and organs receive more oxygen-rich blood. Your blood arteries close off when you're submerged in ice water, making your heart work harder to pump blood. Your cardiovascular system can be strengthened by making an extra effort, which will enhance oxygenation and circulation in general. Additionally, the cold water can aid in lowering blood vessel inflammation, which can improve blood flow and lower your risk of heart disease. It's crucial to remember, though, that anyone with pre-existing heart issues should consult a doctor before undergoing cold water therapy.

How Cold Water Therapy Can Help Repair Your Body and Speed Up Recovery

Cold water therapy can hasten the healing process of an injury or help you recuperate from a strenuous workout. The healing of damaged tissues may be aided by the reduction of edema and inflammation brought on by the cold water. The delivery of essential nutrients and immune cells to the wounded area can be aided by cold water therapy, which can also assist to stimulate blood flow and oxygenation. It's important to keep in mind nevertheless that cold water therapy shouldn't take the place of qualified medical attention. If you have an accident or medical problem, you should always seek medical advice.

. . .

COLD WATER THERAPY has a number of physical advantages that can help you feel better physically and more in general. Cold water therapy is a potent weapon in your wellness toolbox, helping to reduce inflammation and pain, improve circulation, and speed up healing. However, it's crucial to keep in mind that cold water therapy is not a universal cure and might not be appropriate for everyone. Before beginning cold water therapy, always speak with a medical professional, especially if you have any underlying medical concerns. it, go ahead and leap into the chilly waters without hesitation, but do it with care and prudence. Your body will appreciate it!

mental resilience and cold water therapy

. . .

How It Can Improve Your Mood and Boost Your
Energy Levels

THERE ARE several mental benefits associated with cold water therapy, including improved mood and increased vitality. Take a deep breath and join me in plunging into the refreshing depths of mental fortitude!

Improving Psychological Stability with Cold Water Therapy

IT'S easy to feel like you're drowning in life's difficulties when you're up against them. Mental resilience can be strengthened with cold water therapy, making it easier to deal with the stresses of daily life. The release of cortisol and adrenaline, the body's "stress hormones," occurs when you submerge oneself in cold water. You can build up your ability to deal with stress and hardship as a result of this experience. In addition to building mental toughness, completing a cold water immersion can increase one's sense of accomplishment and self-worth.

Maintaining Concentration and Increasing Energy Through Cold Water Therapy

Do you lack energy and motivation? The use of cold water has been shown to increase alertness and productivity. Adrenaline and noradrenaline are released when you submerge yourself in cold water, which can raise your heart rate and rev up your metabolism. If you follow these steps, you may find that you have more energy and are more productive. The cognitive benefits of cold water include increased focus and cognitive ability due to increased blood flow to the brain.

How Cold Water Therapy Can Help Your Mental Health to Conquer Anxiety and Depression

COMMON MENTAL HEALTH issues that might be challenging to manage include anxiety and despair. Anxiety and depression have natural and holistic treatments, and cold water therapy is one of them. Endorphins are released when you submerge yourself in cold water, and these chemicals can help lift your mood and lessen your anxiety and despair. Immersion in cold water has other benefits, including a reduction in ruminating and negative self-talk and an increase in mindfulness. Keep in mind that cold water treatment is not a substitute for seeing a mental health expert. If you're feeling anxious or depressed, it's important to talk to a doctor.

COLD WATER THERAPY has a number of positive effects on the mind that might boost health. Cold water therapy is an effective weapon in the fight against disease and improving your overall health and well-being. Keep in mind that cold water treatment isn't a panacea for mental health issues and shouldn't take the place of seeing a trained specialist. If you are having any mental health issues, you should always seek professional help. Therefore, go headfirst into the chilling depths of mental fortitude. You owe it to your brain.

cold water therapy for sleep quality

. . .

Tips for Better Rest and Relaxation

ARE you sick and weary of tossing and turning in bed, unable to get asleep or stay asleep? If you're having trouble sleeping, a cold shower could be the solution. Taking a cold shower or bath before bed is a tried and true method for relieving stress and improving sleep quality. Let's talk about how cold water treatment can help you get to sleep and how to work it into your nightly routine.

Reducing Stress: The Benefits of Cold Water Therapy Before Bed

IT MIGHT BE CHALLENGING to relax and get to sleep when stress and anxiety are present. Stress and anxiety can be reduced and sleep can be made more restful with the help of cold water therapy. The release of cortisol and adrenaline, the body's "stress hormones," occurs when you submerge oneself in cold water. Dopamine and serotonin, hormones that induce calm and relaxation, are not produced until after you get out of the chilly water. Relaxing in this way helps set the stage for a good night's sleep.

How Cold Water Therapy Can Help You Get Better Sleep by Regulating Your Body Temperature

THE DEGREE to which your body temperature affects the quality of your sleep cannot be overstated. A more restful night's sleep may be the result of a cold water therapy session. Submerging in cold water causes your body's core temperature to drop, which in turn triggers a response to keep warm. This reaction can help your body cool down, making sleep more comfortable. The act of warming up after a dip in cold water can also help your body temperature stabilize, which can improve the quality of your sleep.

How Cold Water Therapy Can Boost Sleep Architecture and Help You Get a Better Night's Rest

THE STRUCTURE OF YOUR SLEEP, including the duration of each stage, is a major factor in the overall quality of your slumber. The structure of your sleep may be enhanced by cold water therapy, leading to better rest. Immersing yourself in cold water causes a stress response, which in turn releases growth hormone and other healing substances. These hormones have been shown to improve sleep quality, particularly the duration and depth of sleep. In addition to enhancing the quality of your sleep, the feeling of being immersed in cold water can shorten the amount of time it takes you to nod off.

THERE ARE several ways in which cold water therapy might enhance the quality of one's slumber. Cold water treatment is a safe and effective technique to get a better night's sleep for a number of reasons, including the fact that it helps you relax, keeps you at a comfortable temperature, and improves the structure of your sleep. Don't be scared to try adding cold water therapy to your nightly regimen. Keep in mind that cold water therapy may not be appropriate for everyone, especially those with certain health conditions. If you have any preexisting medical conditions, you should talk to your doctor before trying cold water therapy. Keeping these considerations in mind will lead to greater sleep and enhanced health.

how to safely integrate cold water therapy into your fitness routine

. . .

DO you want to improve your workouts by adding cold water therapy? The benefits to your body and mind from adding cold water treatment to your fitness program are numerous. But it's important to include cold water therapy properly to avoid damage and maximize benefits. Let's take a look at how you can safely use cold water treatment into your workouts.

Incorporating Cold Water Therapy into Your Workout Routine: A Step-by-Step Guide

To AVOID INJURY, those unfamiliar with cold water therapy should ease into it gradually. Start by taking cold showers or baths after each workout, and work your way up to ice water. You can start introducing cold water immersion into your workouts and training as soon as you feel ready to do so. Keep in mind that cold water therapy isn't for everyone and might not be healthy for those who already have health issues. If you have any preexisting medical conditions, you should talk to your doctor before trying cold water therapy.

Staying Hydrated While Using Cold Water Therapy as Part of Your Exercise Routine

WHEN INCORPORATING cold water therapy into a fitness routine, it is essential to drink enough water. Dehydration can occur due to the quick loss of body heat that occurs after an immersion in cold water. It is essential to drink enough of water before and after undergoing cold water therapy to avoid being dehydrated. Keeping yourself from becoming dehydrated is another important goal of any workout or training session. However, sugary or caffeinated drinks should be avoided because of their diuretic impact, which can lead to dehydration.

How to Hear Your Body and Stay Safe While Exercising in Cold Water

WHEN INCORPORATING cold water treatment into your exercise program, it is essential to pay attention to your body. If you're already tired or nursing an ailment, a cold water plunge may be too much for your body to handle. Pay heed to your body and stop if it tells you to stop doing something. To get the most out of cold water treatment, it's best to ease into it and gradually increase the amount of time spent in the water. This method can assist avoid harm and guarantee the best outcomes.

THERE ARE numerous positive effects of including cold water treatment in your regular exercise program. But it's important to include cold water therapy properly to avoid damage and maximize benefits. Adding cold water therapy to your workout in a safe and effective way is possible if you take it easy at first, drink enough of water, and pay attention to your body. So, dive right in and incorporate cold water treatment into your workout routine. You'll feel better physically and mentally.

the wim hof method

. . .

The Fundamentals of Cold Water Therapy and
Its Benefits

DO you feel prepared to advance your cold water therapy routine? The Wim Hof Technique is the way to go. This technique, developed by Wim Hof, is a combination of cold water therapy, breathing exercises, and meditation. In this section, we'll learn the basics of the Wim Hof Method and how it can improve your health.

Introduction to the Wim Hof Method

THE WIM HOF METHOD is a system of complementary medicine that includes the use of cold water therapy, breathing exercises, and meditation. The theory behind it is called hormesis, and it holds that mild stress can have a beneficial effect on human health. The Wim Hof Method is an approach to improving one's health and happiness that involves immersing oneself in cold water, doing breathing exercises, and meditating.

The Science Behind the Health Benefits of Wim Hof's Cold Water Therapy

THE WIM HOF METHOD relies heavily on cold water therapy. Submerging oneself in cold water has been linked to numerous health advantages. Immersion in cold water has been shown to increase blood flow, decrease inflammation, and strengthen the immune system. Further, it can help you think more clearly and stay strong even when things go tough.

The Science Behind and Benefits of Wim Hof's Breathing Exercises

BREATHING exercises are another component of the Wim Hof Method that can aid in achieving calm, concentration, and clarity of thought. The technique is a series of regulated breathing exercises that have been shown to alleviate stress and anxiety, facilitate relaxation, and boost mental acuity. Breathing exercises provide other benefits, including lowering the risk of chronic stress and its associated health issues through regulating the autonomic nervous system.

Wim Hof Method Meditation: The Science Behind It and Its Health Benefits

THE WIM HOF METHOD relies heavily on meditation to facilitate the desired states of calmness, concentration, and clarity. Meditation has been shown to have positive effects on mental health, including lowering cortisol levels, increasing serenity, and enhancing focus and memory. In addition, meditating regularly helps strengthen one's emotional fortitude, making one less vulnerable to mental health issues like depression.

The Positive Effects on Your Body from the Wim Hof Method

INCREASED BLOOD FLOW, less inflammation, and enhanced immunity are just some of the physical health benefits you can expect to get from practicing the Wim Hof Method. The approach can also help with post-workout recovery and pain management. The Wim Hof Method is an all-encompassing strategy for improving one's health that includes cold water therapy, breathing exercises, and meditation.

Wim Hof's Method and Its Positive Effects on Mental Health.

THE WIM HOF METHOD also has numerous psychological advantages. Reduce stress and anxiety, boost mood, and lessen vulnerability to depression and other mental health problems with this approach, which emphasizes relaxation, mental clarity, and emotional resilience. In addition, the technique can lead to increased introspection and mindfulness, both of which contribute to better health.

Warnings & Cautions Regarding the Wim Hof Technique

THE WIM HOF METHOD has been shown to have positive effects on both physical and mental health, but it must be practiced with care to avoid injury. People with health problems like high blood pressure or diabetes should avoid getting into cold water. Incorrect usage of the method's breathing exercises can lead to dizziness and even hyperventilation. If you have any preexisting medical concerns, it is very important to take a cautious approach to the Wim Hof Method and get a doctor's approval before getting started.

THE WIM HOF METHOD, which incorporates cold water therapy, breathing exercises, and meditation, provides a holistic approach to improving health on all fronts. The Wim Hof Method has been shown to have numerous health benefits, including the promotion of relaxation, mental clarity, increased circulation, decreased inflammation, and enhanced immunological function. Approaching the procedure with prudence and safety in mind is essential, especially if you have any preexisting medical concerns. The Wim Hof Method has the potential to be a game-changer for health and fitness if used correctly. Don't be reluctant to give it a shot and experience the positive effects it has on your body and mind.

combining cold water therapy with other holistic health practices

. . .

Meditation, Yoga, and More

WHY NOT MIX it with other activities for holistic health, like yoga, meditation, and more? In this chapter, we'll look at how combining cold water treatment with other practices can increase its benefits and lead to the best possible health and happiness.

The Power of Cold Water Therapy and Other Holistic Health Practices

ALL HOLISTIC HEALTH TECHNIQUES, like cold water treatment, meditation, yoga, and others, have the same goal: to improve your physical and mental health. By putting these practices together, you can boost the benefits of each one and make a more complete plan for promoting health and happiness.

Combining Cold Water Therapy and Meditation

MEDITATION IS a strong way to clear your mind, calm down, and strengthen your emotions. Meditation can help increase the effects of cold water treatment when done with it. Immersion in cold water can help you feel relaxed and clear-headed, and meditation can help you rest and think more clearly. Also, combining cold water treatment with meditation can help people become more self-aware and mindful, which is good for their general health.

The Benefits of Cold Water Therapy and Yoga

YOGA IS a way to take care of your body and mind as a whole. It includes physical poses, breathing routines, and meditation. When mixed with cold water treatment, yoga can help in many ways to improve both physical and mental health. Immersion in cold water can increase blood flow and lower inflammation, while yoga can make you more flexible, improve your balance, and make you stronger. The mix of cold water therapy and yoga can also help people relax and clear their minds, which can reduce worry and anxiety.

Cold Water Therapy and Breathwork

BREATHWORK IS a natural health practice that includes controlled breathing exercises to help relax, focus, and clear your mind. When mixed with cold water therapy, breathwork can help make the benefits of both methods even better. Immersion in cold water can help you breathe deeper and improve your lung capacity. Breathwork can help you relax and clear your mind. When cold water treatment is combined with breathing exercises, the body's autonomic nervous system can be regulated. This lowers the risk of ongoing stress and the health problems that come with it.

Cold Water Therapy with Massage

MASSAGE IS an approach to health that looks at the whole person. It includes moving soft muscles to help people feel more relaxed, less pain, and better circulation. When massage is combined with cold water treatment, the effects of both can be increased. Immersion in cold water can reduce swelling and improve blood flow, and massage can help you rest and ease muscle strain. Also, combining cold water therapy with massage can speed up recovery after exercise, reduce the chance of injury, and improve total physical performance.

Cold Water Therapy and Nutrition

NUTRITION IS a general health practice that includes eating foods that are high in nutrients to improve health and well-being. Nutrition can help increase the effects of both cold water treatment and eating right. Immersion in cold water can help digestion and nutrient absorption, and eating right can boost immune function, lower inflammation, and improve general health. Also, a mix of cold water treatment and good nutrition can boost energy and improve brain function, lowering the risk of fatigue and health problems that come with it.

Safety Considerations

COMBINING cold water treatment with other natural health practices can be helpful in many ways, but it's important to be careful and safe when doing so. Some techniques, like massage and yoga, can be physically hard and may not be right for everyone. Also, it's important to talk to a medical worker before combining cold water treatment with other methods, especially if you already have health problems. With the right care and direction, however, mixing cold water treatment with other holistic health practices can be a powerful and all-around way to improve health and fitness.

COMBINING cold water treatment with other holistic health practices like meditation, yoga, breathwork, massage, and nutrition can boost the benefits of both practices and support good physical and mental health. But it's important to be careful and safe when doing these things, especially if you already have health problems. With the right care and help, though, you can build a holistic approach to health and fitness that uses the power of cold water treatment and other methods. So, don't be afraid to try different things until you find the right mix of routines for you and your needs.

cold water therapy for enhanced immune system

. . .

How It Can Boost Your Body's Defenses

ARE you seeking for a method to strengthen your immune system that is both natural and efficient? There is no better treatment than ice water therapy! In this chapter, we will investigate the data that supports the claim that a cold water treatment session may strengthen your body's natural defenses and help prevent you from a variety of illnesses.

An Explanation of the Relationship Between the Science of Cold Water Therapy and the Immune System

THE IMMUNE SYSTEM is a complex network of cells and tissues that work together to defend the body against dangerous pathogens like viruses and bacteria. It does this by producing antibodies, which are proteins that bind to and neutralize infections. It has been demonstrated that treatment with cold water can improve the function of the immune system, leading to a stronger and more effective defense against illness.

The role that white blood cells play in the process by which cold water therapy strengthens the immune system

WHITE BLOOD CELL generation and activity are both boosted by cold water therapy, which is one of the ways in which this treatment strengthens the immune system. These cells are in charge of locating and eliminating foreign invaders, such as viruses and bacteria, that have made their way into the body. The use of cold water treatment has been demonstrated to boost the formation of white blood cells as well as their activity level, which results in a more robust immune response.

The connection between anti-inflammatory treatment with cold water and healthy immune function

WHEN THE IMMUNE system detects a threat, such as an infection or damage, it will respond by triggering inflammation. However, prolonged inflammation can cause the immune system to become compromised, which in turn increases the likelihood of contracting a sickness or disease. It has been demonstrated that treatment with cold water can reduce inflammation, leading to both a stronger immune system and a lower chance of developing health disorders that are associated to inflammation.

The use of cold water therapy has been shown to improve immune function, resulting in a lower incidence of illness and disease.

THE COLD WATER therapy can help defend against a variety of illnesses and diseases by improving the function of the immune system. These illnesses and diseases include the flu, the common cold, and even more serious ailments such as cancer. In addition, treatment with cold water can shorten the amount of time needed to recover from an illness and lessen the intensity of its symptoms.

The Relationship Between Stress and Immune Function, as Determined by Cold Water Therapy

THE IMMUNE SYSTEM's inability to operate properly and the associated health issues are both significantly exacerbated by stress. The use of cold water treatment has been demonstrated to lower stress levels, which in turn promotes a better immune system and lowers the risk of health problems associated to stress.

Safety Concerns and Cautionary Measures Regarding the Use of Cold Water Therapy on the Immune System

IT IS essential to approach the practice of cold water treatment with caution and safety in mind, despite the fact that the therapy can give a variety of benefits for the immunological function. Immersion in ice-cold water can be a strenuous physical activity, and it's possible that not everyone should do it. Before beginning a practice of cold water therapy, it is essential to discuss the procedure with a qualified medical practitioner, particularly if you have a history of a medical problem that requires ongoing treatment.

Boosting Your Immunity with Cold Water Therapy: Some Suggestions and Ideas for You to Consider

IF YOU ARE interested in enhancing your immune function with cold water treatment, there are a number of techniques and tactics that you can utilize to make the practice more successful while also making it more pleasurable. Incorporating deep breathing exercises to promote relaxation and mental clarity, employing visualization methods to increase the immune-boosting effects of the practice, and gradually building up your tolerance to cold water immersion are some of the things that may be done.

COLD WATER TREATMENT is a method that is both effective and natural in boosting immune function and promoting general health and wellness. The use of cold water treatment has been shown to help defend against a wide variety of illnesses and disorders, as well as promote faster recovery and decreased symptoms. This is accomplished by boosting the formation and activity of white blood cells; lowering inflammation; and reducing stress levels. However, it is crucial to approach the practice with caution and safety in mind, particularly if you have pre-existing medical concerns. Keeping these in mind will help ensure that you have a positive experience. Cold water treatment has the potential to be a strong tool for strengthening immunological function and overall well-being, provided that it is administered with the appropriate level of care and supervision.

understanding the risks
of cold water therapy and
how to avoid them

. . .

THE USE of cold water treatment is an efficient method for enhancing both one's physical and mental health; yet, like to any other technique, it does include certain inherent dangers. In this chapter, we will discuss the possible dangers of cold water treatment as well as the preventative measures that may be taken.

A Comprehensive Look at the Dangers of Cold Water Therapy, Including Hypothermia and the Cold Shock Response

HYPOTHERMIA and a cold shock reaction are the two most significant dangers that are connected with cold water treatment. In severe circumstances, mortality can result from hypothermia, which is caused when the core temperature of the body drops below normal levels. Symptoms of hypothermia include disorientation and tiredness. The cold shock reaction is a reflex response that is generated when an individual is exposed to cold water. This response can produce an involuntary gasp and increase the danger of drowning.

Exposure to Cold Water Should Be Done Gradually, and the Right Gear Should Be Used So That You Don't Get Hypothermia.

IT IS vital to progressively build up your tolerance to cold water immersion over the course of time in order to reduce the danger of developing hypothermia when undergoing cold water treatment. In addition, using the appropriate gear, such as a wetsuit or neoprene socks, can assist in keeping your body warm and lessen the likelihood of developing hypothermia.

Controlled breathing and a safe entry are two key components in preventing cold shock response during cold water therapy.

DURING COLD WATER TREATMENT, it is essential to ease into the water gradually and in a risk-free manner, practicing regulated breathing methods to prevent uncontrollable gasping, and minimizing the danger of experiencing a cold shock response. In addition, training in safe entrance procedures, such as the "seal entry," can assist in lowering the probability of experiencing a cold shock response.

Other Potential Dangers of Cold Water Therapy Include Pre-Existing Health Problems as Well as Poor Water Quality

EVEN THOUGH HYPOTHERMIA and the cold shock response are the principal dangers linked with cold water treatment, there are still additional possible dangers that should be considered. People who already have certain medical disorders, such as coronary artery disease or asthma, may have an increased probability of experiencing difficulties as a result of receiving cold water treatment. In addition, drinking polluted water increases your risk of becoming sick or getting an infection.

Cold water therapy should only be performed after consulting a qualified medical professional and following all applicable safety procedures.

It is vital to contact with a healthcare practitioner before commencing the practice of cold water therapy in order to limit the risk of damage or disease associated with the treatment. This is especially crucial if you have any pre-existing medical issues. In addition, practicing safe behaviors, such as gradually building up your tolerance to cold water immersion, utilizing adequate equipment, and staying away from sources of water that may be polluted can help lower the chance of damage or sickness.

Cold water therapy is an effective method for improving both one's physical and mental health; yet, it is essential to be aware of and take precautions against any possible hazards that may be linked with the practice. The principal hazards associated with cold water treatment are hypothermia and the cold shock reaction; however, these risks can be minimized by gradually increasing exposure, using the appropriate equipment, and practicing safe entrance procedures. In addition, those who have pre-existing medical issues should speak with a healthcare expert prior to commencing a practice of cold water therapy, and practitioners of cold water therapy should take care to avoid polluted water sources. You may safely and successfully implement cold water therapy into your health and wellness regimen if you first recognize the potential dangers of this technique and then take steps to mitigate or eliminate those dangers.

making cold water therapy a lifestyle

. . .

Incorporating It into Your Daily Routine

YOU ARE NOT ALONE IF, after experiencing the advantages of cold water treatment, you are interested in incorporating it into your daily routine on a more consistent basis. In this chapter, we will discuss some suggestions and techniques for implementing cold water therapy into your lifestyle so that you may continue to gain the mental and physical health advantages associated with this practice.

Beginning on a Small Scale Will Help You Build Your Tolerance

IF YOU HAVE NEVER USED cold water treatment before, it is essential to begin slowly and progressively increase the amount of time you spend in the cold water as your tolerance increases. Start by taking cold showers for a few seconds at the end of your usual shower, and gradually increase the length of time you spend under the cold water until you are showering for the whole recommended period of time. It is crucial to take your time and pay attention to your body as you build up your tolerance to cold water. Eventually, you may be able to work up to complete immersion in a chilly pool or body of water, but until then, you should take baby steps.

Establish a Schedule for Yourself and Keep to It

It is essential to establish a regimen and stay committed to it if you want to make cold water treatment a consistent component of your way of life. Make your cold water therapy practice a top priority in your agenda and select a consistent time and location for it to take place on a regular basis. You will have a better chance of maintaining your cold water treatment regimen over time if you approach it as a non-negotiable component of your daily routine.

Improve the quality of the experience by practicing various breathing and visualization techniques

Increasing the advantages of cold water treatment while also making the experience more pleasurable can be accomplished by using strategies including visualization and breathing. Imagine that you are courageous and able right before you step into the icy water, and concentrate on your breathing to help you settle your thoughts and get your body ready. Maintain your composure and ease throughout the cold water immersion by practicing some deep breathing exercises.

To Speed Up Your Recovery, Apply Warm Water and Practice Warming Techniques

It is imperative that, following a session of cold water treatment, efforts be taken to bring the body back up to temperature and facilitate recovery. try introducing warming routines such as stretching or a warm cup of tea into your routine, and try using hot water to warm up your body and boost circulation first. In addition, make sure that you drink enough of water and eat well to aid in the process of your body getting well.

Don't Forget the Benefits of Cold Water Therapy on Your Mental Health!

Although it is more often known for its positive effects on one's physical health, cold water treatment also has significant positive effects on one's mental health. The use of cold water treatment as part of a person's regular practice can help alleviate stress and anxiety, raise mental clarity and focus, improve mood, and increase energy levels.

Including cold water treatment into your daily routine on a consistent basis may be a potent tool for enhancing both physical and mental wellness when done so regularly. You may make cold water treatment a fun and sustainable part of your lifestyle by beginning with a little amount, establishing a pattern, including visualization and breathing exercises, and starting small. In addition, remember the significance of healing, as well as the significant positive effects that this practice has on one's mental health. You may continue to reap the benefits of cold water treatment by keeping the aforementioned suggestions and tactics in mind, and you can also make it a regular part of your routine for maintaining your health and fitness.

zero to hero

. . .

Economical 30-Day Plan for Embracing Cold
Water Therapy

ARE you considering integrating cold water therapy into your daily routine? This economical shift doesn't require high-end equipment or a large budget. It's all about making a simple yet significant lifestyle tweak. With this in mind, let's get started!

Cold water therapy, often underestimated, is a powerhouse of benefits. It's a natural energy booster, like a shot of espresso but without the caffeine jitters. When you step into that cool cascade, your heart rate increases, blood flow improves, and you'll feel invigorated, ready to tackle the day.

It also fortifies your immune system. Imagine your body as a fortress; cold water therapy strengthens the walls, making it harder for diseases to invade. Regular exposure to cold water increases the production of white blood cells, your body's soldiers against illness.

Moreover, it improves skin and hair health. Warm water can strip away natural oils that keep your skin and hair moisturized. Cold water, on the other hand, helps to seal in these oils, leaving your skin glowing and your hair shining. Consider it a free spa treatment right in your home!

Now, if you're worried about the discomfort, rest assured, it's easier than you might imagine. The human body is a marvel of adaptability. Just like it learns to wake up at the same time every morning or adjust to a new pair of glasses, it can accustom itself to cold water showers. It's all about gradual change, taking it one day at a time.

REMEMBER, you're not aiming for a polar plunge right off the bat. You'll start slow, gradually introducing your body to cooler temperatures. And before you know it, you'll be relishing your daily cold showers.

So, here's your chance to embrace an economical, straightforward shift with abundant health benefits. Cold water therapy is not just a trend; it's a lifestyle change that can significantly boost your well-being. It's all about taking that first step, and with each passing day, you'll find it easier than you thought. Ready to give it a try?

Day 1-7: Testing the Waters

START by introducing your body to the cool sensation gradually. Don't think of it as a shock, but rather as a friendly hello from a new acquaintance. Begin your regular showers with your usual warm temperature. Then, for the last 30 seconds, turn the knob towards the cooler side. You don't need to go ice-cold just yet; a moderate chill will do. Keep reminding yourself, like a mantra, that it's just a little discomfort for a boatload of benefits.

Day 8-14: The Cool Down

By now, your body should be getting accustomed to the new routine. Let's turn it up a notch. Extend the cool down period of your showers to a minute or two. Try to breathe calmly and think of something that makes you happy. Picture yourself as a seasoned hiker, embracing the chilly mountain air.

Day 15-21: The Plunge

You're halfway through your journey, and it's time to truly embrace the cold. Start your shower with a lukewarm temperature and then go full cold for the last three to five minutes. Yes, it will be challenging, but remember, you're a resilient mountain hiker, and this is just another hill to climb.

Day 22-30: The Icy Regimen

You've made it to the final stretch! It's time to kick it into high gear. Try starting your shower at a lukewarm temperature and switch to cold halfway through. Maintain the cold temperature for the rest of your shower. You're not just a hiker now; you're a mountain climber, conquering the icy peaks!

.   .   .

Keep in mind; consistency is key. Make it a part of your daily routine and stick to it, like a dedicated artist working on a masterpiece.

Now, let's talk nominal expenses. A shower timer could be a useful tool to keep track of your progress. You can find an affordable one online or at a local store. This will help ensure you're sticking to your plan and increasing your cold exposure as intended.

Another small investment would be a journal to record your experiences. Note down how long you spent in the cold water each day, how you felt during and after the shower, and any changes you notice in your body or mood over time. This will not only track your progress but also motivate you to keep going.

Remember, safety first. Listen to your body. If you ever feel dizzy or overly uncomfortable, it's okay to step back and warm up. The goal is to challenge yourself, but not at the cost of your well-being.

In this 30-day plan, you're not just making a small change in your daily routine; you're making a significant leap towards a healthier lifestyle. So, here's to you, soon-to-be cold water therapy pro. Your journey may be chilly, but the benefits you reap will be warmly rewarding!

conclusion

. . .

YOU SHOULD at this point be aware of the benefits of cold water therapy as a potent technique that has a number of advantages for both one's physical and mental health. Cold water treatment has the ability to alter your health and wellness routine in a variety of ways, including the reduction of inflammation and discomfort, as well as the promotion of mental clarity and focus.

IN THIS BOOK, we have covered a variety of topics, including the science behind cold water therapy and its numerous advantages, as well as advice and tactics for getting started with the practice, becoming an expert at it, and incorporating it into your daily routine. Before beginning a practice of cold water treatment, it is essential to confer with a medical expert and go over any potential dangers, as well as how to prevent them. This topic has been covered extensively throughout this article.

. . .

IT IS essential to approach the art of cold water treatment with the utmost reverence and caution, regardless of whether you are a novice or an experienced practitioner. It is possible to lessen the likelihood of suffering an accident or becoming unwell if you prepare for exposure to cold water in stages, make sure you have the right gear, and practice safe entrance procedures. Incorporating visualization and breathing methods, as well as taking efforts to warm up and recuperate after a session of cold water treatment, can boost the advantages of the practice and make it more pleasurable overall.

THE CAPACITY of cold water therapy to strengthen mental fortitude and foster an optimistic frame of mind is one of the most potent characteristics of this treatment modality. We cultivate a feeling of mental fortitude and acquire a sense of resilience when we put ourselves through the mental strain of enduring the discomfort of cold water immersion. This sense of fortitude and resilience may then be applied to other aspects of our lives. In addition, the use of cold water treatment can assist in the alleviation of stress and anxiety, the promotion of relaxation and peaceful sleep, as well as an improvement in mood and levels of vitality.

IT IS possible to further improve the advantages of cold water therapy by combining it with other holistic health activities such as meditation, yoga, and breathwork. While cold water therapy is a strong practice in its own right, it may also be paired with these other disciplines. We can construct a strong arsenal for enhancing both our physical and mental health as well as building resilience in our lives by integrating cold water therapy with other disciplines and creating a hybrid of the two.

IT IS vital to approach cold water treatment with care and respect since it has the potential to be a life-changing event, but it must first be incorporated into your daily routine. Cold water therapy is a powerful tool that may help you accomplish your health and wellness objectives. You can use it to improve your physical performance, reduce pain and inflammation, or boost mental clarity and focus. All of these benefits can be achieved by utilizing cold water therapy.

I WANT to encourage you to look into the field of cold water treatment and learn more about the numerous advantages that it can provide. You have the ability to alter your health and wellness via the power of cold water, whether you do it by having a cold shower in the morning, leaping into a cold pool, or practicing the Wim Hof Method. Take the risk, learn to tolerate the discomfort, and you'll be able to access the numerous advantages that this potent practice has to offer.

bonus: beyond cold showers

. . .

A Comprehensive Guide to the Wim Hof
Method and Its Benefits

Unlock your full potential with our 3-chapter bonus from
the companion book:

Beyond Cold Showers: A Comprehensive Guide to the
Wim Hof Method and Its Benefits

By: Hunter Hazelton

Hunter Hazelton

BEYOND
COLD
SHOWERS

A Comprehensive Guide to the
Wim Hof Method and Its Benefits

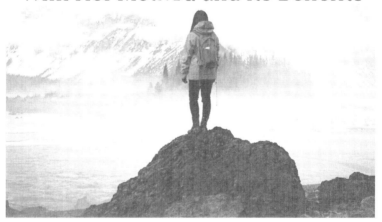

discovering the wim hof method

. . .

A Path to Extraordinary Health

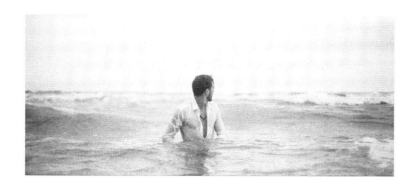

Meet Wim Hof: The Ice Man

LET'S dive into the frosty world of Wim Hof, the man who defied the laws of nature and transformed his life through cold exposure and controlled breathing. Known as the Ice Man, Wim Hof has dedicated his life to helping others unlock their potential and achieve optimal health, proving that the seemingly impossible is within reach. As we explore the life and achievements of this extraordinary individual, you'll discover how his unique method can revolutionize your life, too.

BORN in the Netherlands in 1959, Wim Hof's journey began with a simple curiosity that led him to experiment with icy waters. His connection to the cold started when he was just 17 years old, as he took his first plunge into a frozen pond. This experience ignited a spark within him, leading to a lifetime of exploration and discovery in the realms of mind and body.

THROUGHOUT HIS LIFE, Wim Hof continued to develop his unique approach to cold exposure and controlled breathing. Over the years, he has broken multiple world records, including climbing Mount Kilimanjaro and Everest wearing only shorts, swimming under ice, and completing a full marathon in the Namib Desert without drinking water. His incredible feats of endurance and mental strength have attracted the attention of both the media and the scientific community, further fueling the curiosity surrounding his method.

WIM HOF's ability to withstand extreme cold and control his body's physiological responses can be attributed to his deep understanding and mastery of his own breath. Through a combination of cold exposure and controlled breathing, he has developed a method that enables individuals to tap into their innate power and enhance their physical and mental well-being. The Wim Hof Method has since gained popularity worldwide, attracting a diverse range of followers seeking to improve their health, boost their immune system, and achieve peak performance.

AS YOU DELVE DEEPER into the life of Wim Hof and explore his groundbreaking method, you'll find that it's not just about facing the cold. It's also about embracing the power of the mind and harnessing its potential to overcome physical and mental barriers. Wim Hof believes that the mind, body, and soul are interconnected, and through the practice of his method, one can achieve a harmonious balance that leads to improved health and overall well-being.

IT's essential to remember that Wim Hof's success isn't solely based on his exceptional abilities. Instead, he is driven by an unwavering determination to challenge conventional wisdom and push the boundaries of human potential. His passion for self-discovery and exploration has led him to develop a method that can truly benefit everyone, regardless of age or background.

．　．　．

THE STORY OF WIM HOF, the Ice Man, serves as a testament to the power of human will and resilience. By daring to push the limits and embrace the unknown, he has unlocked the door to a world of possibilities that awaits those willing to take the plunge. As we continue to explore the Wim Hof Method, we'll delve into the science behind this extraordinary practice, unraveling the mysteries that surround cold exposure and controlled breathing. In doing so, we'll discover how understanding the science behind the method can provide the foundation for you to embark on a transformative journey, ultimately enhancing your health and empowering you to achieve the seemingly impossible.

Understanding the Science Behind the Method

DELVE into the fascinating world of the science behind the Wim Hof Method, a revolutionary practice that has transformed countless lives by tapping into the body's natural potential. By understanding the underlying principles of this method, you'll be equipped with the knowledge to harness the power of cold exposure and controlled breathing, enabling you to overcome mental and physical barriers and reach new heights.

THE WIM HOF METHOD primarily revolves around two key elements: cold exposure and controlled breathing. Cold exposure works by stimulating the body's natural response to cold temperatures, causing a series of physiological changes. For instance, when the body is exposed to cold, blood vessels constrict, resulting in increased blood flow and circulation. This response has been shown to improve immune function, reduce inflammation, and enhance overall health.

MOREOVER, cold exposure activates the body's natural production of brown adipose tissue, also known as brown fat. Unlike white fat, which stores energy, brown fat generates heat and burns calories. Studies have found that individuals with higher levels of brown fat tend to have faster metabolisms, making it easier for them to maintain a healthy weight and reduce their risk of developing metabolic disorders.

CONTROLLED BREATHING, the second pillar of the Wim Hof Method, focuses on optimizing the body's oxygen levels to improve overall health and performance. By engaging in deep, rhythmic breathing, you can increase the amount of oxygen in your blood, which in turn enhances cellular respiration and energy production. This practice also stimulates the release of endorphins, promoting feelings of happiness and well-being while reducing stress and anxiety.

ONE OF THE most significant aspects of the Wim Hof Method is its impact on the autonomic nervous system, which regulates essential functions such as heart rate, digestion, and respiratory rate. Traditionally, it was believed that the autonomic nervous system could not be consciously controlled. However, Wim Hof's remarkable achievements and the subsequent scientific research have demonstrated that with the right techniques, individuals can indeed influence their autonomic nervous system.

A GROUNDBREAKING STUDY conducted by Radboud University in the Netherlands provided evidence supporting the benefits of the Wim Hof Method. Participants who practiced the method showed a significant increase in their ability to withstand cold temperatures and reported a decrease in inflammation markers. Furthermore, the study revealed that these individuals could voluntarily activate their sympathetic nervous system, a feat previously thought to be impossible.

WHILE THE WIM HOF METHOD is rooted in science, it's essential to recognize that it is not a one-size-fits-all solution. Each individual's response to the method may vary, and it's crucial to listen to your body and adapt the practice to your unique needs and limitations. By doing so, you'll be able to experience the full potential of this transformative method, ultimately leading to improved health, resilience, and performance.

AS WE CONTINUE to explore the Wim Hof Method, it's vital to address the myths and misconceptions that may arise. By debunking these misconceptions, we'll shed light on the true nature of the method and empower you to make informed decisions as you embark on your journey toward optimal health and well-being. So, buckle up and get ready to uncover the truth behind the Wim Hof Method, a practice that has the power to revolutionize your life and unlock your full potential.

Debunking Myths and Misconceptions

IT's time to separate fact from fiction and debunk myths and misconceptions surrounding the Wim Hof Method. By dispelling these inaccuracies, you'll be better equipped to embrace the benefits of this transformative practice, empowering you to unlock your full potential and enhance your physical and mental well-being.

A COMMON MISCONCEPTION about the Wim Hof Method is that it's reserved for the fearless and the physically elite. The reality, however, is that this practice is accessible to anyone willing to step outside their comfort zone and explore their body's innate capabilities. While it's true that some individuals, such as Wim Hof himself, have taken the method to extreme levels, the core principles can be adapted to suit the needs and limitations of each individual.

ANOTHER MYTH IS that the Wim Hof Method is purely a cold exposure practice, with some believing that simply taking cold showers or ice baths is all that's required. Although cold exposure is a significant component of the method, controlled breathing and mindset training play equally important roles in achieving the desired outcomes. It's the synergy of these three elements that allows practitioners to reap the full benefits of the Wim Hof Method.

SOME SKEPTICS MAY ARGUE that the Wim Hof Method is nothing more than a placebo effect, with the power of belief driving the positive results. However, numerous scientific studies have validated the efficacy of the method, demonstrating its impact on the immune system, inflammation, and the autonomic nervous system. These findings provide substantial evidence that the Wim Hof Method goes beyond mere placebo and has a genuine effect on the body and mind.

IT'S ALSO worth addressing the misconception that practicing the Wim Hof Method is dangerous or risky. While there arc inherent risks associated with cold exposure and breath-holding exercises, these can be minimized by following proper guidelines and listening to your body. It's crucial to build up your tolerance gradually and avoid pushing yourself beyond your limits. By doing so, you can safely harness the power of the Wim Hof Method without jeopardizing your health.

LASTLY, some people may believe that the Wim Hof Method is a cure-all solution to a wide range of health issues. While the method has been shown to improve various aspects of health, it should not be considered a substitute for medical advice or treatment. It's essential to view the Wim Hof Method as a complementary practice that can enhance your overall well-being and work in tandem with conventional medical care.

Now that we've dispelled these myths and misconceptions, it's time to dive deeper into the world of the Wim Hof Method and explore the myriad benefits it has to offer. In the upcoming section, we'll delve into the transformative effects of this practice on both your body and mind. From boosting your immune system to enhancing mental clarity, you'll soon discover how the Wim Hof Method can revolutionize your life and set you on a path towards optimal health and happiness. Get ready to embrace the power within you and unlock your full potential as we continue this exhilarating journey.

Embracing the Benefits: Physical and Mental Well-being

Once you understand the remarkable benefits of the Wim Hof Method and its impact on physical and mental well-being you might just think you uncovered a secret of the universe. By embracing this transformative practice, you'll unlock a world of possibilities, enhancing your overall health and empowering you to reach new heights in both your personal and professional life.

· · ·

A CORNERSTONE of the Wim Hof Method's physical benefits lies in its ability to strengthen the immune system. Cold exposure and controlled breathing work in tandem to stimulate the body's natural defenses, making it more resilient to illness and infection. Studies have shown that individuals who practice the Wim Hof Method exhibit increased white blood cell production and reduced inflammatory markers, equipping them with a more robust immune response.

BEYOND IMMUNE FUNCTION, the Wim Hof Method has been found to improve cardiovascular health. By exposing the body to cold temperatures, blood vessels constrict and then dilate, promoting better circulation and oxygen delivery to vital organs. This process can lead to increased energy levels, reduced fatigue, and enhanced endurance, making it easier for practitioners to tackle daily tasks and challenges.

THE WIM HOF METHOD's controlled breathing exercises also play a crucial role in physical well-being. By increasing oxygen levels in the bloodstream, these exercises promote optimal cellular function, facilitating more efficient energy production and helping the body perform at its best. This heightened state of oxygenation can also contribute to faster recovery from physical exertion and improved athletic performance.

IN ADDITION to its physical benefits, the Wim Hof Method boasts a host of mental health advantages. One of the most notable effects is its ability to alleviate stress and anxiety. The controlled breathing exercises help activate the parasympathetic nervous system, which is responsible for the body's relaxation response. By tapping into this calming state, practitioners can experience reduced stress levels, lower blood pressure, and a greater sense of overall well-being.

MOREOVER, the Wim Hof Method has been shown to enhance mental clarity and focus. The combination of cold exposure and controlled breathing exercises can increase the release of endorphins and other neurotransmitters, which are crucial for maintaining a positive mood and sharp mental acuity. This boost in cognitive function can lead to better decision-making, heightened creativity, and improved problem-solving skills.

THE WIM HOF METHOD's impact on mental well-being also extends to fostering resilience and mental fortitude. By challenging the body and mind to overcome the discomfort of cold exposure, practitioners develop a more robust mindset, enabling them to face life's obstacles with greater courage and determination. This newfound sense of inner strength can translate to increased confidence and self-esteem, further fueling personal and professional growth.

AS WE CONTINUE to learn more about the wonders of the Wim Hof Method, we'll shift our focus to the power of oxygen and its role in our bodies. In the next section, we'll uncover the science behind controlled breathing and its profound effects on our physical and mental health. From optimizing energy production to promoting relaxation, prepare to be amazed by the incredible potential that lies within each breath.

breathing to energize

. . .

Mastering the Wim Hof Breathing Technique

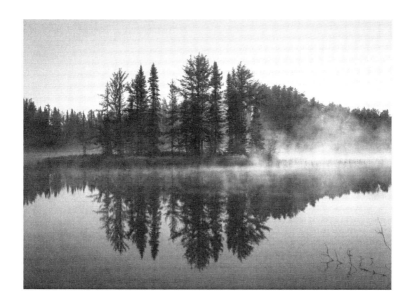

The Power of Oxygen: How Breathing Affects Your Body

AT THE HEART of the Wim Hof Method's effectiveness lies the incredible role of oxygen in our bodies. Oxygen is a vital component in the production of adenosine triphosphate (ATP), the primary source of cellular energy. With every breath we take, we fuel our cells with the necessary resources to perform countless tasks, from muscle contractions to brain activity.

WHEN WE PRACTICE CONTROLLED breathing exercises, like those found in the Wim Hof Method, we can optimize oxygen intake and enhance our body's ability to generate energy. By taking slow, deep breaths, we allow more oxygen to enter our bloodstream and reach our cells, leading to more efficient energy production and improved overall function.

IN ADDITION to its impact on energy levels, proper oxygenation can have profound effects on our mental health. Oxygen plays a crucial role in maintaining a healthy brain, as it helps regulate the production and release of neurotransmitters, such as serotonin and dopamine. These chemicals are essential for promoting a positive mood, reducing stress, and enhancing focus. By engaging in controlled breathing exercises, we can ensure our brain receives the optimal amount of oxygen it needs to function at its best.

. . .

ANOTHER FASCINATING ASPECT of oxygen's role in our bodies involves its connection to the autonomic nervous system. This system, responsible for regulating many of our body's automatic functions, is divided into two branches: the sympathetic nervous system (SNS) and the parasympathetic nervous system (PNS). The SNS is responsible for activating our "fight or flight" response during times of stress, while the PNS helps us enter a more relaxed, "rest and digest" state.

BREATHING IS something we do every day without giving it much thought. But what if I told you that the simple act of focusing on your breath could bring about a wide range of health benefits? The Wim Hof Method, a set of breathing exercises, is here to show you how.

The Wim Hof Method revolves around controlled breathing exercises that aim to balance the parts of our nervous system responsible for rest and action. You see, our body's autonomic nervous system has two main parts: the sympathetic nervous system (SNS) and the parasympathetic nervous system (PNS). The SNS is in charge of our "fight or flight" response, while the PNS helps us "rest and digest." In our fast-paced world, it's common for the SNS to be overactive, leaving us feeling stressed and on edge.

THAT'S where the Wim Hof Method comes in. By focusing on slow, deep breaths, we can activate the PNS and tell our brain it's time to relax. The result? A whole host of positive changes in our body, like less anxiety, lower blood pressure, and better digestion.

You might be wondering, "How exactly does the Wim Hof Method work?" Well, the process is simple but powerful. It involves taking a series of deep breaths in and then exhaling without forcing the air out. After doing this several times, you hold your breath on the last exhale for as long as you can. Finally, you take a big breath in and hold it for a short time before returning to normal breathing.

When you practice these exercises regularly, you'll start to notice that your body and mind feel more balanced. For example, people who use the Wim Hof Method often report feeling calmer and more focused throughout the day. And because a relaxed mind is closely linked to a healthy body, many users also notice improvements in their physical well-being.

But the benefits don't stop there. The Wim Hof Method is also known to help with sleep. Having trouble falling asleep or staying asleep is often a result of an overactive SNS. By using the breathing exercises to activate the PNS, you can calm your body and mind, making it easier to drift off into a peaceful slumber.

The Wim Hof Method can even support a stronger immune system. Studies have shown that regular practice can lead to a decrease in inflammation, which is a key factor in many health issues, including chronic pain and autoimmune diseases. By keeping inflammation in check, the Wim Hof Method can help your body stay healthy and better equipped to fight off illness.

THE BEAUTY of the Wim Hof Method is that it's accessible to everyone, regardless of age, fitness level, or experience with breathing exercises. All it takes is a commitment to practice and an openness to the transformative power of the breath.

AS YOU CONTINUE to use the Wim Hof Method, you may find that it becomes an essential part of your daily routine. Many people look forward to their breathing sessions as a way to center themselves and prepare for the day ahead or unwind after a long day.

THE IMPACT of the Wim Hof Method on overall well-being cannot be understated. By tapping into the power of controlled breathing, you can unlock a world of benefits that ripple out into every aspect of your life. From reduced stress and improved sleep to better digestion and a stronger immune system, the potential gains are vast and varied.

PERHAPS ONE OF the most intriguing aspects of the power of oxygen is its ability to boost our body's innate healing processes. When our cells have access to an optimal supply of oxygen, they can more effectively repair damaged tissues and fend off potential infections. This heightened state of healing can contribute to faster recovery from injuries, reduced inflammation, and a stronger immune system.

Step-by-Step Guide to the Wim Hof Breathing Technique

THE WIM HOF BREATHING TECHNIQUE revolves around three main components: deep inhales, passive exhales, and breath retention. Begin by finding a comfortable position, either sitting or lying down, where you can fully relax and focus on your breath. Ensure that you are in a safe environment, as the technique may cause lightheadedness.

ONCE SETTLED, initiate the process with a series of deep, diaphragmatic breaths. Inhale through your nose, filling your lungs to their maximum capacity. Visualize the air flowing down into your diaphragm, allowing your belly to expand outward. This deep breathing helps maximize oxygen intake and stimulate the body's natural relaxation response.

FOLLOWING EACH DEEP INHALE, let the air flow out of your lungs effortlessly through your mouth. Avoid forcefully exhaling or holding your breath. Instead, allow your body to release the air naturally, without any tension or strain. This passive exhale enables your body to release carbon dioxide and maintain a healthy balance of gases within your bloodstream.

· · ·

CONTINUE the cycle of deep inhales and passive exhales for approximately 30 to 40 breaths, or until you start to feel a tingling sensation in your extremities. This sensation is a sign that your body is ready for the next phase: breath retention.

UPON COMPLETING YOUR FINAL EXHALE, pause and hold your breath for as long as you comfortably can. This breath retention phase allows your body to further absorb oxygen and release carbon dioxide, promoting a state of deep relaxation and enhanced focus. As you hold your breath, remain calm and composed, observing any sensations or thoughts that arise.

WHEN YOU FEEL the urge to breathe again, take one more deep inhale, filling your lungs completely. Hold this breath for approximately 15 seconds before releasing it slowly through your mouth. This final inhale and brief retention serve as a "recovery breath," allowing your body to re-establish its equilibrium.

REPEAT the entire process for two to four more rounds, or as long as you feel comfortable. With each cycle, you may find yourself able to hold your breath for longer periods, further enhancing the technique's benefits.

Tips for Proper Technique and Avoiding Common Mistakes

SELECTING an appropriate location is crucial to the success of your practice. Find a quiet, comfortable space free from distractions, ensuring you have ample room to breathe and stretch. Whether indoors or outdoors, the environment should encourage relaxation and focus, setting the stage for a productive session.

MAINTAINING proper posture is equally important, as it enables you to breathe deeply and efficiently. Regardless of whether you're sitting or lying down, ensure your spine is in a neutral position, with your head, neck, and shoulders relaxed. Avoid slouching, as this can restrict airflow and hinder the effectiveness of your practice.

WHILE THE WIM HOF BREATHING TECHNIQUE may be intense, it's essential to listen to your body and respect its limits. If you experience dizziness or lightheadedness, don't push yourself too hard. Instead, pause for a moment and resume the practice at a slower pace or with less intensity. Remember, your well-being should always come first.

CONSISTENCY IS the key to achieving lasting benefits from your breathing practice. Make a commitment to regular sessions, ideally setting aside time each day for focused practice. This consistency will allow you to develop and refine your technique while fostering a deeper connection with your breath.

. . .

ONE COMMON MISTAKE is holding the breath for too long, which can result in unnecessary strain and discomfort. Instead, aim for a comfortable duration that allows you to experience the benefits of breath retention without compromising your well-being. With time and practice, your ability to hold your breath will naturally improve.

TO MAXIMIZE the effectiveness of your breathing practice, synchronize it with other aspects of your daily routine, such as meditation or exercise. By integrating your practice into a holistic approach to well-being, you'll create a synergistic effect that amplifies the benefits of each individual component.

ANOTHER CRITICAL ASPECT TO consider is your mindset. Approach your breathing practice with a curious and open mind, free from judgment or expectation. This attitude will allow you to fully immerse yourself in the experience and gain deeper insights into your breath and its impact on your body and mind.

Tailoring Your Breathing Practice for Optimal Results

BEGIN by identifying your specific objectives and intentions for your breathing practice. Are you looking to reduce stress, boost energy levels, or improve focus and concentration? By clarifying your goals, you'll be better equipped to design a personalized practice that addresses your unique needs and aspirations.

It's essential to consider your individual preferences and lifestyle when designing your breathing practice. Factors such as your daily schedule, preferred practice environment, and physical limitations can all play a role in determining the most effective approach for you. By taking these factors into account, you'll create a practice that seamlessly integrates with your life and yields maximum results.

Experimentation is a crucial aspect of tailoring your breathing practice. Be open to trying different techniques and approaches, monitoring their impact on your body and mind. By paying close attention to how various practices affect you, you'll gain valuable insights that inform your ongoing customization process.

Incorporating complementary practices, such as yoga, meditation, or mindfulness, can further enhance the benefits of your breathing practice. By combining these disciplines, you'll create a synergistic effect that amplifies the advantages of each component while fostering a holistic approach to well-being.

Don't be afraid to make adjustments to the duration, intensity, and frequency of your practice as needed. Remember, your needs may change over time as your body and mind evolve. By staying attuned to your shifting requirements and adapting your practice accordingly, you'll maintain a dynamic and responsive routine that continues to serve you well.

It's ALSO important to recognize that your breathing practice may require different approaches depending on your current physical and emotional state. For example, if you're feeling anxious or overwhelmed, you may benefit from a calming technique, such as diaphragmatic breathing. Conversely, if you're seeking to boost your energy levels or focus, a more invigorating practice, like the Wim Hof Breathing Technique, may be more suitable.

REMEMBER that consistency is key to achieving lasting benefits from your breathing practice. Establish a regular practice schedule, setting aside dedicated time each day for focused sessions. By making your breathing practice a non-negotiable aspect of your daily routine, you'll foster the discipline and commitment necessary for long-term success.

DEVELOPING A DEEPER understanding of your breath and its impact on your body and mind will also aid in your customization efforts. By educating yourself on the science and mechanics of breathing, you'll be better equipped to make informed decisions about which techniques and approaches are best suited to your needs.

DON'T HESITATE to seek guidance and support from experienced practitioners or experts in the field of breathwork. By tapping into their knowledge and insights, you'll gain valuable perspective and inspiration that can help you refine your practice and overcome any challenges that may arise.

ONE OF THE most critical aspects of tailoring your practice is remaining open to change and evolution. As you progress on your journey, your needs and goals may shift, necessitating adjustments to your approach. By staying flexible and open-minded, you'll ensure that your practice continues to serve you well throughout every stage of your personal growth journey.

cold exposure

. . .

Unleashing Your Inner Warrior

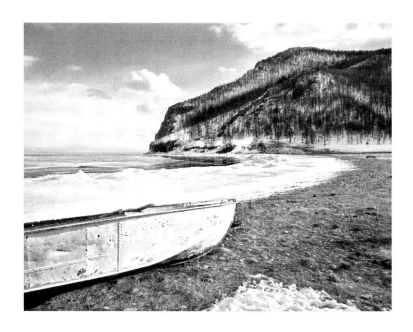

The Science of Cold Therapy: Boosting Your Immune System

COLD THERAPY, also known as cryotherapy, has long been recognized for its ability to reduce inflammation and improve circulation. When the body is exposed to cold temperatures, it activates a series of physiological responses that help regulate the immune system. These responses include increased white blood cell production, which plays a vital role in defending the body against infections and disease.

IN ADDITION to enhancing immune function, cold therapy has been shown to stimulate the release of endorphins, also known as "feel-good" hormones. This flood of endorphins can help improve mood, reduce stress, and increase overall feelings of well-being. By incorporating cold therapy into your wellness routine, you'll not only support your immune system but also promote emotional balance and resilience.

ANOTHER KEY BENEFIT of cold therapy lies in its ability to activate brown adipose tissue, also known as brown fat. Unlike white fat, which stores excess energy, brown fat generates heat and burns calories. By stimulating brown fat through cold exposure, you can boost your metabolism and support weight management.

. . .

As YOU EXPLORE the science of cold therapy, it's important to remember that every individual is unique, and what works for one person may not work for another. Always listen to your body and consult with a healthcare professional before beginning any new health regimen, especially if you have existing medical conditions or concerns.

IF YOU'RE new to cold therapy, start by learning about various techniques and approaches, such as cold showers, ice baths, and cryotherapy chambers. By familiarizing yourself with these methods, you'll be better equipped to determine which approach best aligns with your goals and preferences.

IT'S ALSO helpful to educate yourself on the science behind cold therapy. By understanding the physiological mechanisms at play, you'll gain a deeper appreciation for the practice and its potential benefits. This knowledge will empower you to make informed decisions about your cold therapy routine and ensure that you're maximizing its positive impact on your immune system and overall health.

As YOU EXPERIMENT with cold therapy, be prepared for some initial discomfort. However, it's essential to distinguish between discomfort and pain. While a certain level of discomfort is normal, it's crucial to listen to your body and never push yourself to the point of pain or injury.

. . .

Remember that consistency is key when it comes to reaping the benefits of cold therapy. Establish a regular practice schedule and commit to it, just as you would with any other wellness routine. Over time, your body will adapt to the cold, and you'll begin to notice improvements in your immune function, mood, and energy levels.

Now that you're equipped with a solid understanding of the science behind cold therapy, it's time to take the plunge and explore the world of gradual exposure. From cold showers to ice baths, you'll learn how to safely and effectively incorporate cold therapy into your daily routine. By taking a measured and mindful approach, you'll unlock the full potential of this powerful practice, bolstering your immune system and fostering a greater sense of well-being.

Gradual Exposure: From Cold Showers to Ice Baths

Embrace the chill and unlock the transformative power of cold therapy by taking a step-by-step journey from cold showers to ice baths. Gradual exposure to the cold is the key to unlocking the full potential of this powerful practice, paving the way for a healthier and more resilient version of yourself.

Starting with cold showers is a great way to ease into cold therapy. The simplicity and accessibility of this method make it an ideal entry point for those new to the practice. To begin, try ending your regular shower with a 30-second burst of cold water. As your body adapts, you can gradually increase the duration and intensity of the cold exposure, eventually working up to a full cold shower.

As you progress with cold showers, you'll likely begin to notice improvements in your mood, energy levels, and overall well-being. These positive changes are a testament to the power of gradual exposure and will serve as a source of motivation as you continue to challenge yourself.

When you're ready to take your cold therapy practice to the next level, consider exploring the world of ice baths. This more intense form of cold exposure offers a range of benefits, including enhanced recovery, reduced inflammation, and improved immune function. However, it's important to approach ice baths with caution and respect, as the extreme temperatures involved can pose risks if not properly managed.

Before diving into an ice bath, it's essential to prepare both physically and mentally. Begin by taking slow, deep breaths to calm your mind and center your focus. This mindful approach will help you maintain control and presence throughout the experience.

When you're ready to immerse yourself in the ice bath, do so slowly and mindfully. Remember that your body will naturally react to the cold with an initial shock response, characterized by rapid breathing and an increased heart rate. Focus on your breath and allow yourself to relax into the experience, acknowledging the discomfort without allowing it to overwhelm you.

As you become more comfortable with ice baths, you can experiment with various techniques and durations to find what works best for you. Some people prefer shorter, more intense sessions, while others may opt for longer, more moderate exposure. The key is to listen to your body and find the balance that maximizes the benefits without causing undue stress or strain.

Throughout your cold therapy journey, it's crucial to remember that consistency is key. Establish a regular practice schedule and commit to it, just as you would with any other wellness routine. By doing so, you'll continue to unlock the full potential of cold therapy, reaping the rewards of improved immune function, enhanced mood, and increased resilience.

As you venture further into the invigorating world of cold therapy, it's important to prioritize safety and best practices. Whether you're a seasoned ice bath enthusiast or just beginning your journey, staying informed and mindful of the risks and precautions associated with cold exposure will ensure that you're able to safely and effectively reap the benefits of this powerful practice.

· · ·

IN THE UPCOMING SECTION, we'll delve deeper into the safety precautions and best practices that are essential for a successful and enjoyable cold therapy experience.

Safety Precautions and Best Practices

EMBARKING on the cold therapy journey can be invigorating and transformative, but it's essential to prioritize safety and adhere to best practices to ensure a rewarding experience. In this section, we'll explore the precautions and guidelines you should follow to make the most of your cold therapy practice while minimizing risk.

ONE OF THE fundamental principles of safe cold therapy is to listen to your body. While it's natural to experience discomfort during cold exposure, it's crucial to differentiate between manageable sensations and those that signal potential harm. If you ever feel lightheaded, dizzy, or experience intense pain, it's important to end the session immediately and warm up.

WHILE ENGAGING IN COLD THERAPY, maintaining a calm and focused mindset is vital. Before each session, take a moment to center yourself and practice deep, controlled breathing. This mental preparation will help you stay present and aware of your body's signals during the cold exposure, allowing you to respond effectively to any sensations or signs of distress.

. . .

WHEN YOU'RE ready to progress from cold showers to ice baths, be cautious and gradual in your approach. Start by immersing only your lower body and gradually work up to full immersion over time. This slow progression will help your body acclimate to the extreme temperatures and minimize the risk of adverse reactions.

ANOTHER ESSENTIAL ASPECT of cold therapy safety is understanding the importance of duration. While longer cold exposure sessions can offer increased benefits, it's crucial to strike a balance between maximizing gains and avoiding overexposure. As a general guideline, aim for sessions lasting between 2-10 minutes, but always defer to your body's feedback and adjust accordingly.

A CRUCIAL CONSIDERATION in cold therapy is the prevention of hypothermia. Make sure to monitor the temperature of your ice baths, and never let the water temperature drop below 50°F (10°C). Additionally, ensure that you have a way to rewarm your body quickly after each session, such as a warm blanket or a heated room.

IT'S ALSO important to be mindful of the environment in which you practice cold therapy. Ensure that the space is free of hazards, such as slippery surfaces or sharp objects, and always have a support system in place. This could be a buddy who joins you in the cold therapy session or someone who remains close by to offer assistance if needed.

. . .

REMEMBER that consistency is key when it comes to cold therapy. Establishing a regular routine and sticking to it will help you safely progress and maximize the benefits of this powerful practice. However, if you ever feel unwell or suspect that you may be coming down with an illness, it's best to pause your cold therapy practice until you recover.

As YOU CONTINUE to hone your cold therapy skills, it's essential to track your progress and celebrate your milestones. In the next section, we'll delve into methods for monitoring your growth and acknowledging your accomplishments, fostering a sense of pride and motivation that will propel you further on your cold therapy journey.

BY KEEPING these safety precautions and best practices in mind, you'll be well-equipped to explore the transformative world of cold therapy with confidence and assurance. As you progress, you'll unlock the full potential of this powerful practice, boosting your immune system, enhancing your well-being, and discovering new depths of resilience and strength.

Tracking Progress and Celebrating Milestones

TRACKING progress and celebrating milestones is more than just a feel-good exercise—it's a vital component in the journey to growing your business and achieving your dreams. In this section, we'll explore the importance of monitoring your growth, acknowledging your accomplishments, and the various techniques that can help you stay motivated and focused on your goals.

ONE POWERFUL WAY TO track your progress is by keeping a detailed record of your achievements and challenges. A dedicated journal, spreadsheet, or digital app can serve as a valuable tool for logging your experiences and reflecting on your growth. By consistently documenting your journey, you'll be better equipped to identify areas for improvement and make informed decisions about the direction of your business.

BUT TRACKING progress doesn't have to be all about numbers and metrics. It's also essential to recognize the personal growth and insights you gain along the way. Pay attention to the lessons you learn, the relationships you build, and the obstacles you overcome. These intangible experiences are just as important as the quantifiable markers of success.

IN ADDITION to monitoring your progress, celebrating milestones is crucial in maintaining motivation and a positive mindset. When you reach a significant goal or complete a challenging project, take the time to acknowledge your hard work and dedication. Whether it's a small victory or a major breakthrough, every accomplishment deserves recognition.

· · ·

CELEBRATIONS CAN BE AS simple or elaborate as you choose. You might want to share your success with friends or colleagues, treat yourself to a special indulgence, or simply take a moment to reflect on your journey so far. The key is to find a way to honor your achievements and reaffirm your commitment to your goals.

ANOTHER POWERFUL MOTIVATOR is sharing your journey with others. Joining a community or networking group can provide invaluable support and encouragement, as well as the opportunity to learn from the experiences of others. Connecting with like-minded individuals who share your passion and drive can help you stay focused and inspired on your path to success.

AS YOU TRACK your progress and celebrate milestones, don't forget to periodically reassess your goals and aspirations. The world of business is dynamic and ever-changing, and it's crucial to remain adaptable and open to new opportunities. By regularly evaluating your objectives and adjusting your course as needed, you'll ensure that you're always moving forward with purpose and intention.

IN THE PURSUIT OF SUCCESS, it's essential to recognize the intrinsic connection between your mind and body. As we transition to the next topic, we'll delve deeper into this profound relationship and explore how nurturing this connection can enhance your overall well-being and propel you towards your goals.

· · ·

By EMBRACING the practice of tracking progress and celebrating milestones, you'll not only gain valuable insights into your journey but also foster a sense of motivation and pride that will fuel your continued growth. Remember, every step forward brings you closer to achieving your dreams and unlocking your full potential. So, keep your eyes on the horizon, celebrate your achievements, and get ready to embrace the transformative power of understanding the connection between your mind and body.

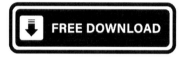
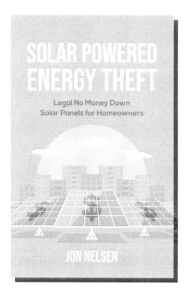

Manufactured by Amazon.ca
Acheson, AB